Table of Contents

- Preface

- Congratulations

- The Unbreakable Bond Between Mental and Physical

- The Five Senses and Sensory Overload

- Establish a Confidant

- Radical Acceptance

- **How to Become Aware of Your Emotions**

- **Stress and Emotions**

- **Adjusting your Lifestyle**

- **DIY Coping Strategies**

- **Seeking Outside Help**

- **References**

Preface

Bend Without Breaking is an amalgam of tribute to those who have struggled with mental health and a memoir of the things I discovered in navigating my illness.

The coping mechanisms outlined here are by no means exhaustive, but they do serve to set you on a path toward mental wellness and hope. For me, I wish this book had existed when I was thrashing about and trying to fight the waves of my disease, as it would have served to provide me with the starting point you will now have.

For you, I hope this book represents the beacon of light you need and helps you to understand one thing if nothing else; if you have already come across this learning, I hope the book serves you as a notification to focus on things that matter the most.

Above all, and no matter what, you will be okay.

Congratulations

I want to begin this book by commending you and simply telling you, *"Congratulations."*

In the world of mental health, the most challenging step is almost always the first one: accepting that you need help.

As humans, we are born with an instilled sense of pride and an innate attitude that not only can we do anything we put our minds to, but we can do it alone. Unfortunately, for many, this causes a certain stigma around mental health that it's something to be ashamed because, more often than not, one must resort to asking for help.

As someone who suffers from chronic anxiety and intermittent depression, trust me when I say I understand how you feel. The word "Help" makes your stomach wraith and twist like a ball of constrictor snakes. You would rather suffer alone for the rest of your life than reach out just once and admit that you can't do this on your own.

Like I said, I understand. And you aren't alone. One in four people worldwide will suffer from mental or neurological issues at some point in their lives, so the fact that you're struggling at this moment is not a testament that you are weak. It is a testament that you are human and that you can feel very deeply.

In short, having to reach out and work on your mental health is not something to be ashamed of. Instead, the exceptional mental health you'll have when you come out on the other side will be a badge you can wear with honour, and that will enable you to help others, given a chance.

Some of the topics you might find helpful, some you feel things could have been the other way around, can take steps from the book, making you happier and merrier.

Do share the ideas/thoughts you learned from this book with the need. Remember, we grow together.

Dhineshsunder Ganapathi

The Unbreakable Bond Between Mental and Physical

To achieve the level of mental wellness that you want, we need to understand how psychological and physical are tied together. You cannot have fitness in only one if the other is out of equilibrium. As such, good mental health begins with taking care of your physical health.

You can think of the brain as a muscle. For your muscles to function when you are working out, they need specific nourishment. Water, for example, and protein. Complex carbohydrates are promising to provide you with energy, and electrolyte-heavy beverages surely wouldn't hurt. Similarly, you need to ensure your brain is fed with everything it needs before you begin working it out to make it stronger. You can make excellent strides in this area by doing the following:

Get 8 Hours of Sleep

I'm sure this is an adage you've heard a million times, but there is some science behind it. Physically, sleep deprivation leaves your brain exhausted, which means it doesn't perform at maximum capacity and resulting in physical consequences, such as lack of coordination and trouble concentrating.

Furthermore, your brain has a more challenging time regulating your body when it doesn't enough time to rest. The disharmony in brain can cause blood pressure fluctuations, increased or decreased heart rate, and feelings of dizziness or vertigo. All of these physical symptoms then have adverse mental health because you become worried and afraid that something is wrong with you when, in reality, you need a nap essential to note in this area that not all people will need 8 hours. Some will require more, and some will need less. Generally, though, the range will be between 7-10 hours, depending on your age. If you are younger (such as in your teens), you could need as much as Eleven or twelve hours because your body is expending so much energy growing.

Drink Enough Water

You saw this one coming. Your trainer would have a fit! After all, how are you supposed to exercise a muscle without adequate hydration?

Not drinking enough can have health effects similar to sleep deprivations, such as regulating bodily functions like heart rate and blood pressure and cause headaches and nausea. In short, not drinking enough water can make you feel physically sick as well as mentally sick.

We need to address one thing in this area: drinking 8 cups of water per day is a myth (unless you play some extreme sports.) When I say drink enough water, drink it when you're thirsty instead of reaching for soda, a coffee, or an energy drink. Even if you're drinking water once in a while, but you should be drinking more water them put together.

Eat a Balanced Diet

Our diet can have a massive effect on our mental health, and no wonder! It's where we receive the bulk majority of our vitamins and minerals for the day, and having a poor diet can have loads of mental health repercussions.

The best thing you can do in this area is to stay away from fast food. It will get you nowhere fast, and studies have shown that fast food can contribute to and cause depression in the brain.

Instead, you want to ensure you're getting enough food to sustain yourself and eat things rich in healthy compounds such as fruits and vegetables. I find strawberries and blueberries to be excellent snacks, and I love making homemade smoothies!

I only have one more tip for you in this area: have your local drug store vitamin supplements. Many vitamins can prompt your body and brain to have more energy and be happier overall, and others can calm you down and help you sleep.

My advice is to purchase a B-vitamin complex supplement as B vitamins are known to provide energy and happiness throughout the day. Additionally, I find L-theanine to be an effective, calmer and healthy, natural sleep agent. It also works well in a pinch when I find myself having a nasty bout of anxiety.

Keep in mind when purchasing supplements that only certain ones are water-soluble (meaning your body will flush out the excess). Others are fat-soluble and can cause issues if you consume too much because your body does eliminate the ones you don't need. In general, A, E, D, and K are the fat-soluble vitamins to stay away from, but you should consult your doctor to see what's right for you.

Not generalizing, but whenever we wanted to take the next steps in our health management, Most often than not, we check on some random YouTube channel/WhatsApp forwards or any other social media junk and blindly following the message. Please don't do it, I beg you, Be conscious of the vitamin supplements you're in, Consult your doctor before hopping into any.

And If you're not comfortable working on consuming vitamin supplements, drop it right away. It's not a hard and fast rule; when it comes to medications and vitamin supplements, be diligent on it and make the right choice

Disclaimer: I am not a medical professional, and this chapter (as well as this book) does not constitute medical advice. Always consult with your doctor before taking a new supplement or following any of these tips.

The Five Senses and Sensory Overload

In coping with mental health, your senses can be both a blessing and a curse. The senses can calm you down from crisis-like situations, or they can cause them. In this chapter, we will teach you to use them to help yourself rather than hurt.

Sensory Overload

Sensory overload occurs in many people with mental health disorders, especially in those with anxiety or depression. It can also be an indicator of certain neurological diseases, such as Autism or ADHD.

The overload usually occurs when you become highly stimulated because your brain begins to have trouble processing all of the signals it is receiving. It can result in feelings of dread, panic attacks, etc.
Sensory overload is often worse when you already have intense thoughts in the back of your mind, taking up the majority of your processing power.

Using Your Senses to Your Advantage

Sensory overload can be incredibly inconvenient, but you can use your senses to stop it the same way you used them to start it.

In situations where you believe you are experiencing sensory overload, you can use the 5-4-3-2-1 method. Using those numbers in that order, you anchor yourself by critically examining your surroundings one sense at a time. To use this technique, say or think the answers to the following:

What are five things you can see?
What are four things you can feel?
What are three things you can hear?
What are two things you can smell?
What one thing you can taste?

The above technique increases or decrease difficulty and take up less or more of your attention and time. By the end of this process, you should begin to feel less anxious and overwhelmed. If you aren't, do it again and keep doing it until you do.

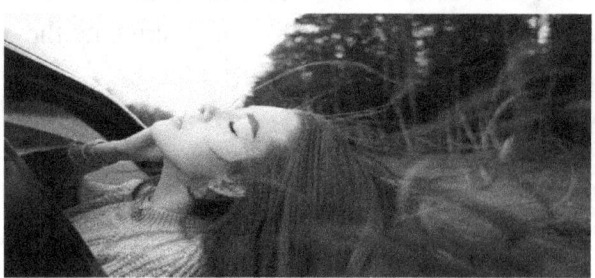

Eventually, you will feel yourself beginning to calm, and your anxieties will slip away.

Is it necessary to note that, while the example listed above is constructive and works for most people, it may not work in certain situations? Why? You feel yourself beginning to panic? It is always best to remove yourself from the case and get to a calmer, quieter area.

I find that hearing too many loud, intermingling sounds at once is the trigger that pushes me over the edge, so I tend to bring earplugs or noise-cancelling headphones to places I know will be loud or hectic always have my earbuds with me just in case. If things ever get too loud unexpectedly, I pop them in and listen to a AR Rahman songs. The method to attain serenity differs people to people, have one in hand always so that you ensure there is a reset/calm button when all hell broke loose. You can also pack provisions when you go out to help decrease the number of times this happens.

Establish a Confidant

As I stated in the first chapter, humans are prideful creatures that think they can manage everything by themselves, including keeping themselves mentally healthy.

Here's a bombshell for you, though: you can't do it alone.

You can practice all the coping skills you like, partake in meditation, and recite countless mantras, but the truth is you need someone else. Humans are social creatures, and having someone to split the burden of mental health with you can improve your progress 10-fold. This confidant can be a friend you enjoy speaking to who you trust not to judge your issues, it can be a diary you pour your thoughts out into, or it can be a therapist.

I highly recommend the third one, as therapists are well-equipped to listen without judging and are required by law not to tell anyone what you tell them. They're personal diaries that provide feedback and reassurance where you need it. They could also likely give you more coping strategies than this book can.

If you can, it is always a good idea to establish multiple confidants that you feel comfortable sharing your feelings. Therapists are excellent for providing coping techniques to you, but they won't give the same comfort that a best friend or significant other could.

When working with a confidant, make sure you're mindful of them and check well before opening with them the Therapists or your friends for the record. This method will ensure that things don't get ugly; when going ahead with the confidant, make sure you trust them completely.

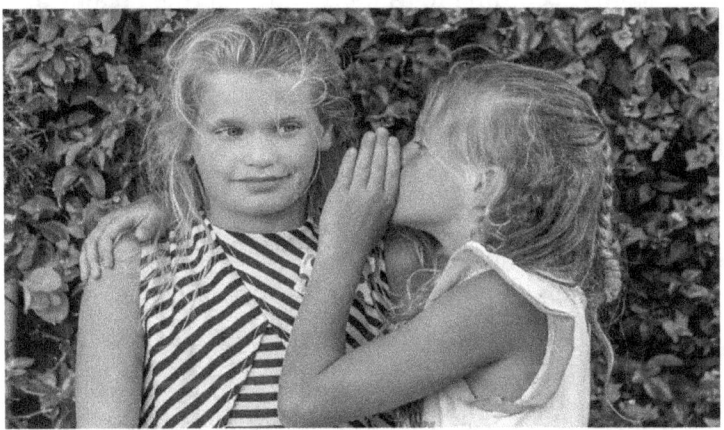

Not to mention, neither of those can provide you with love and care that a parent or grandparent might be able to.

One thing be conscious of the confidant you're choosing, things may go south, If the confidant is trust-worthy

Radical Acceptance

Radical acceptance is likely the most powerful coping mechanism you can have in dealing with mental illness. But, unfortunately, it is the area where most people struggle the most.

Radical acceptance in the mental health field is "completely and accepting something from the depths of your soul," according to Marsha Linehan (the creator of DBT, or Dialectal Behaviour Theory). This principle centres around the idea of accepting the things you cannot change as, once you take them entirely, they begin to cause much less grief.

Think of it like drowning. If you're in the middle of a lake panicking and thrashing in the water because you think that if you stop, you're going to go under, you're going to be terrified to accept the fact that you might drown. However, you'll find that once you acknowledge that you may go under, you calm down. Then, because your body is naturally buoyant, you begin to float.

Mental health works much the same way. If you thrash about and fight against your mind with all your might, you aren't going to get very far. All of that time you spend pretending it isn't there or willing it to go away is just draining you of energy and positive emotions. So instead, accept it as a part of you.

Will it likely one day go away? Yes.

But for now, you must accept yourself the way you are and float on the waves, taking the hits as they come.

Emotional Awareness

With radical acceptance comes a practice is known as emotional awareness. This coping mechanism works off the same principle as the former: if you fight against your emotions, it will take longer to overcome them.

It happens because much like the example with the lake. We need to stop fighting for a moment to analyze our situation. So, if you're feeling depressed or anxious, don't panic. Take a moment to allow yourself to handle all of those emotions and accept them as a part of you. Then, after that moment is over, begin taking action to decrease the emotional turmoil, such as listening to music or reading a book.

The most crucial principle to understand here is that you can control how you feel just by willing yourself not to feel that way.

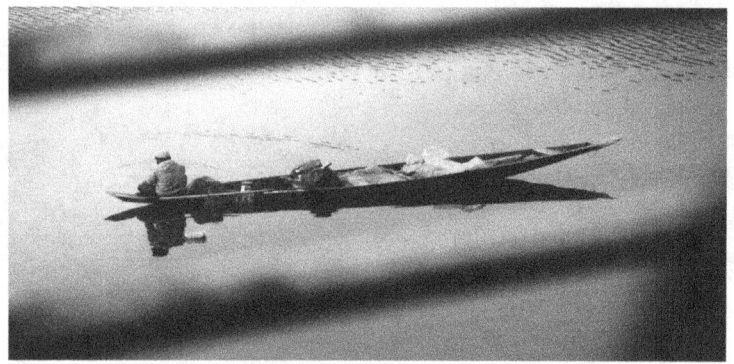

You can, however, control your response to those feelings. As a matter of fact, in doing so, you take power away from your mental illness and give it back to yourself.

Remember one thing, everyone has their flaws, if we accept it, no one can use them against us. There is nothing wrong about it; we are imperfect, and we fail to spot the elephant in the room. Spot it, and plan on the next steps.

How to Become Aware of Your Emotions

When you live in denial of your emotions, you often spend more time repairing and maintaining them. However, once you recognize and accept what you're feeling, you're able to take a step back and analyze your issues and take the steps needed to repair yourself.

One mistake that many people make is exhausting themselves by constantly trying to fight off their unpleasant emotions. If you're feeling anxious and depressed, often the best thing to do is to sit back for a moment and let yourself feel those feelings before you rush into repair mode.

Anxious? Feel it for a moment and then meditate. Angry? Sit with it before listening to some calming music. You can't control how you have to deal with these feelings, but you can control how you react.

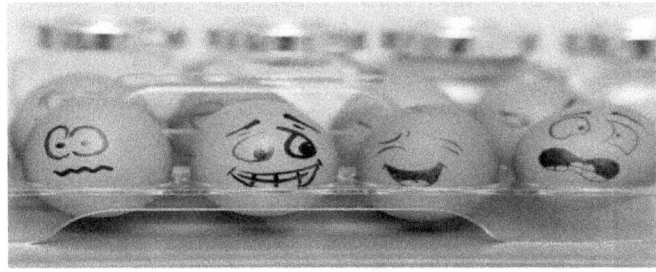

It does take strength and persistence to recover and thrive despite your illness, but that doesn't mean you have to cut it off the moment when the anxiety kicks in.

It is important to remember that these feelings you're having are a part of you, and you need to be gentle with yourself.

Over time, this coping mechanism will help you to establish a healthier way of thinking and managing your issues by getting you into the habit of thinking with your rational brain first and emotions second. This fact alone is enough to make emotional awareness an insanely important method of coping.

Stress and your Emotions

Now that we've discussed how to deal with complex emotions let's, talk about what can trigger them and how to mitigate or avoid those triggers.

Stress is the biggest trigger of mental illness that exists. Unfortunately, stress is caused by nearly anything in our daily lives, even seemingly minor issues. Here is some example of things in your everyday life that can cause stress:

- Being homeless
- Losing your job
- Financial Concerns
- Health Fears
- Being Bullied
- Concerns about family or relationships
- Moving to a new environment
- Having a close family member pass away
- Going to an appointment
- Interviewing for a new job
- Changing your career path

These are just a few events that occur day-to-day that can cause us significant stress. In the world of mental illness, though, we often categorize the pressures we're feeling without realizing it until it manifests in physical or emotional symptoms we don't recognize. These symptoms then cause us to panic focuses more, which leads to more symptoms.

Stress can cause this vicious cycle to continue until you are grossly overwhelmed and have no idea how to stop the spiral. Because of this, the key here is to recognize when you are experiencing symptoms of stress and then try to determine the root cause of those symptoms. The following are some example of symptoms you may experience as a result of stress:

Physical

- Headaches
- Unusual Sweating
- Vertigo
- Muscle Tension
- Dizzy Episodes
- Fast Heartbeat
- Trouble Breathing
- Dry Mouth

- Heart Palpitations
- Stomach Problems
- Muscle Aches and Pains

Mental

- Catastrophizing (assuming the absolute worst will happen based on no objective evidence)
- Forgetting things
- Constant worrying
- Unusual irritability
- Racing thoughts
- Making mistakes
- Unable to concentrate
- Feeling sad for no reason

Behavioural

- Crying
- Change in appetite
- Nail-biting
- Shivering
- Avoiding socialization
- Insomnia

- Hypersomnia
- Increase in drinking or smoking
- Unusual snappiness

As you can see, there are dozens of issues that stress can cause, and there are even hundreds more than this. Because of this, it's essential to recognize the signs of tensions within your own body so you can address the issue and mitigate the symptoms.

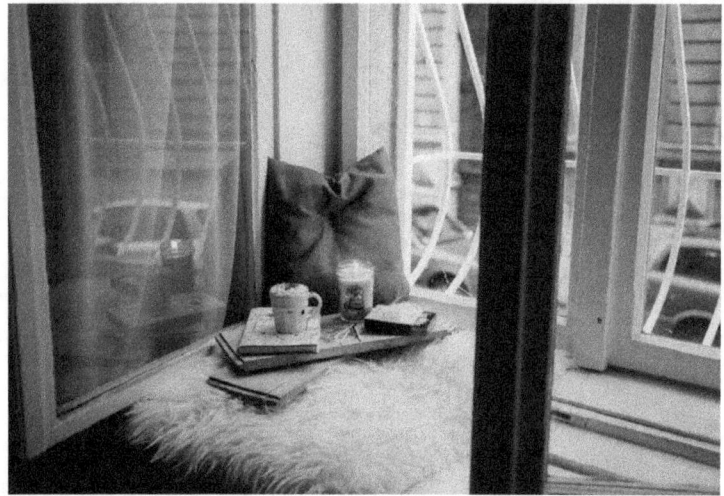

So, once you've identified the issue, how does it self-soothe for you so that it causes less anguish?
There are a few ways:

Stress Diary or Bullet Journal:

Often, the first step to overcoming the stress and pain it is causing is to get it out. You can do this by talking to your confidant or establishing a stress diary or bullet journal. Often, it's more helpful to do both.

Once you put those worries and stresses onto paper, your brain recognizes that it can now begin to let them go because those concerns are stored elsewhere. This activity allows you to focus more on the things that please you and less on those that don't.

A bullet journal, on the other hand, has a variety of applications. It helps us to track your exercise, water intake, mood, spending, and dozens of other things. It is helpful because it assists you in establishing a routine and setting goals, which makes you feel more in control. As a result, that thing is stressing you start to matter much less. In spending or worrying about your health, you are also taking active steps to eliminate the problem, thereby solving your stress two-fold.

Note: Both of these techniques function as hobbies that serve to take your mind off of your issues and are incredibly effective coping mechanisms.

Address the Issue

The second step to eliminating your pain point is to address the issue at hand. Are your concerns financial? Are you related to housing? Relationship-based? Whatever it is, it's a good idea to seek out practical advice.

To do this, target somewhere that can give you advice on your problem in particular (therapists are great, and everyone should have one, but they can't always give you the practical advice you need).

For example, if your issues are financial, discuss with your significant other or a financial advisor how to cut down expenses. Additionally, you can also read free eBooks and online courses on establishing additional income streams.

For those with housing-related issues, visit your local housing authority and talk to them about reduced-cost or income-based housing. You can also look for accommodation in your area or (in very urgent scenarios) visit your local homeless shelter, so you have a bed for the night.

Some shelters will also allow you to stay for days, weeks, or months so long as you are actively looking for employment or work.

As you can see, there are plenty of professionals who are qualified to help your situation. The most important thing you can do is to find them.

Focusing on your Lifestyle

Everyone has stress, problems and their own bottlenecks to ponder over, but what makes us unique is how we react to it. If we are able to maintain our calm during tedious/dreadful situations, we win. I drew inspiration from MS Dhoni, A veteran cricketer for India, The way he maintains his calm during dire situation, earns his name **CAPTAIN COOL** At the end of the day, It's not about winning or losing, It's how we handle the situation. We will win and lose n number of times in our life, it depends on multi-variant factors, but keeping the compose, will redefine us.

My two cents for reducing (and possibly eliminating) your stress is to make necessary lifestyle changes , which we will address in next chapter

Adjusting your Lifestyle

Lifestyle changes materially material things that act upon the body to reduce stress and increase emotional tolerance. By making these adjustments, you increase your ability to be flexible with difficult situations.

Limit Caffeine

Caffeine is a stimulant that works to speed up both your body and mind, the latter of which precisely is exactly favourable in dealing with stress. Products such as coffee, chocolate, energy drinks, and certain types of tea all contain caffeine. Therefore, missing your intake could help you manage day-to-day difficulties better and help you sleep better.

If you have to have the energy, I recommend trying out B-vitamin supplements to provide yourself with natural, long-lasting energy without the negative consequences. Also, if you love the taste of coffee, decaf will be your best friend.

Exercise Regularly.

Not only does exercise help you keep your body healthy, but it also functions to keep your mind running smoothly as well. For example, in exercising, you make it harder to obsess over the things you are afraid of by tiring out both your body and mind so that neither have the energy to stress and panic.

Exercise also releases chemicals in the brain, such as dopamine and endorphins, known to have lasting health benefits and promote happiness and calm.

Get Enough Sleep

I have stressed this in my first chapter, why eight hours of sleep is important for your mental health, It also helps as a mechanism to cope up stress. Getting enough sleep can often be difficult, especially if you struggle with managing stress. However, if you aren't getting the recommended amount of stress, it can lead to several negative impacts such as poor concentration, mood swings, and low emotional stability. These problems only get worse the more sleep you lose.

If sleep is something you struggle with, you can try to help yourself wind down by putting away your phone an hour before bedtime, as the blue light your phone emits can cause your brain not to release those chemicals that kick in and make you sleepy. You can also try things like exercising more during the day and avoiding caffeine past about noon.

If you have tried these things and nothing seems to work, though, there are other strategies you can try:

● First, discuss your issue with your doctor. Ask about supplements that may help you wind down, such as melatonin or L-theanine.

● Second, establish a regular bedtime routine so that your body and brain both recognize when it is time to go to sleep.

● Make sure the place you sleep is dark and not too hot. By cooling the temperature in your bedroom, you lower your core body temperature, which signals to your brain that it is time to sleep.

● It would help if you only were lying in your bed when you intend to sleep. It allows your brain to recognize that you should be going to sleep the moment you lay down.

● Journal or read just before bed, as both of these things allow your brain to a particular singular activity, rather than running wild and thinking about what you're doing tomorrow, what you did that day, or whatever else you tend to think about when trying to fall asleep.

- Keep a notepad by your bed to essential important thoughts that occur to you as you're falling asleep, so you don't obsess over possibly forgetting them and can let them go.

- Finally, some people need a certain amount of white noise to fall asleep. If you have trouble sleeping, I recommend keeping a small fan in your room to move air around and provide white noise to help lull you into dreamland.

Practice Self Care

Perhaps the most crucial part of adjusting your lifestyle to reduce stress and promote healthy thinking is practising good self-care. By allowing yourself to do or experience things that make you happy, you encourage a better disposition within yourself.

I recommend doing at least one nice thing for yourself every day. It could be something like soaking in a bubble bath, going out for your favourite coffee, or eating food you love.

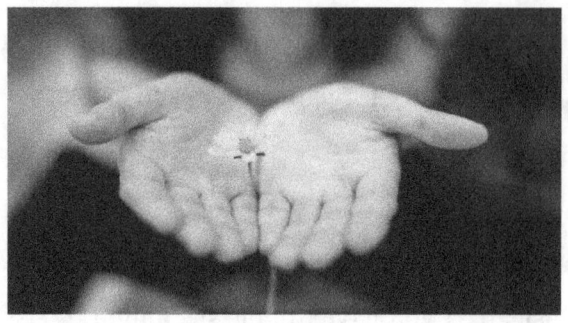

Partake in Mindfulness and Relaxation

Mindfulness is a mindset that prioritizes being aware and actively participating in the current moment. It helps deal with stress, anxiety, and depression as it encourages not to consider all the possibilities of what could go wrong but rather what is going right at that moment.

Relaxation techniques help develop this mindset and slow down those rampaging thoughts. Some examples of relaxation techniques can be aromatherapy, meditation, or yoga.

Regardless of your mental illness or its severity, the tips outlined in this chapter will help you adjust your mindset so that you can better focus on being in the present moment.

DIY Coping Strategies

Within this chapter, you'll find a list of coping strategies that I have found helpful throughout my years of coping with anxiety and depression. Some of these may be appropriate for you, and others may not. Similarly, some of them work better in response to emotionally stimulated episodes, and some of them work better in response to problem-stimulated attacks. There will be some trial and error as you figure out what works best for you.

List of Strategies

1. Exercise (walk, run, go to the gym, play Wii Fit)
2. Write your feelings down.
3. Scribble, doodle, or draw
4. Paint
5. Socialize
6. Watch a TV show
7. Restore your old furniture
8. Have a good cry
9. Go shopping
10. Take a hot shower or bath.

11. Go swimming (relaxing in the summer, invigorating in the winter)
12. Clean something
13. Start or complete a sewing project.
14. Bake
15. Reorganize your room/home
16. Meditate
17. Write a letter to your future self.
18. Create a time capsule and bury it in the backyard to dig up a month or year from now
19. Complete that project you've been putting off
20. Contact a therapist
21. Go to your local animal shelter and volunteer or pet the animals.
22. Go for a slow bike ride.
23. Play a video game
24. Take a hike through nature.
25. Drive to your nearest waterfall and take some pictures. If you're feeling bold, go for a swim at the bottom of it (make sure it's safe and allowed!)
26. Sunbathe

27. Go to the library. Once there, either read something or sit among the stacks and appreciate where you are
28. Play Sports
29. Join Toastmasters, network with like-minded people
30. Go for a quick walk to ground yourself.
31. Take a time out and count slowly to ten.
32. Learn a new subject (It can be anything from how rubber bands are made to the history of sunblock, it's up to you!)
33. Practice affirmations in the mirror
34. Cook and eat a healthy snack
35. Jog in place
36. Set some goals to accomplish using the rule of 10: a plan you can achieve within 10 minutes, do within 10 hours, and one within ten days.
37. Colour in a colouring book
38. Walk through the craft's section at Walmart/malls and pick out an activity.
39. Play a new board game with some friends

40. Put together a puzzle from beginning to end. If you're feeling it, get some mod podge and stick it on a piece of cardboard or wood so you can hang it on the wall!
41. Watch a movie you've meant to watch
42. Do something you used to enjoy as a kid but haven't had the chance to do in a while (such as blowing bubbles!)
43. Run carelessly through a field of wildflowers
44. Go on a day trip to the zoo.
45. Go on a date night with your significant other
46. Have a fun time thrift shopping
47. Take a day trip to your nearest amusement park or theme park.
48. Make a list of things you want or need for your house. It can be anything from new furniture to organization containers to a fluffy plush blanket. Then, select a few items and buy them!
49. If you aren't concerned about finances, order a few things online. I know I always get excited to have packages coming!

50. Find a relaxation app that you enjoy. I recommend the app, Antistress.
51. Create a to-do list for yourself for the day, week, and month.

Coping strategies that distract and soothe you are incredibly effective for overcoming the negative emotions associated with mental illness. Of course, there are many more coping strategies than these, but this list will serve as an avenue to get you started and provide you with some healthy and fun activities to partake in the meantime.

Seek Outside Help

This book should have given you a solid basis to build your healthy coping strategies up, but it can't substitute the benefits that a therapist can provide you. Coping strategies tend to tide you over while you work on the core thoughts that cause your mental illness and rewire your brain, so those thoughts no longer cause issues. However, they cannot replace professional help.

Cognitive Behavioral Therapy (CBT) is something many therapists use to readjust how their clients think to help them achieve a healthier, happier life. I highly recommend consulting a therapist about this form of reflective reasoning.

Lastly, I have included the number of helplines at the end of this book. Some of them you have to call but others you can text, as I know how hard it can be to speak over the phone sometimes.

I wish you all the best on your journey and good luck. I know you can do it.

Help Lines:

Suicide Prevention Hotline: 800-273-8255

Anxiety/Depression Crisis Text Line: Text CONNECT to 741741

Mental Health and Substance Abuse Hotline: 1-800-662-4357

Domestic Violence Support Hotline: Call or Text START to 1-800-799-7233

India Suicide and Stress Helpline: Call 1800-233-3330 or email help@jeevanaastha.com.

For any queries, reach out to me at dhineshsunder93@gmail.com.

www.ingramcontent.com/pod-product-compliance
Lightning Source LLC
Chambersburg PA
CBHW081706220526
45466CB00009B/2892